RENAL DIET COOKBOOK FOR BEGINNERS

Simple and Delicious Recipes Low in Sodium, Potassium, and Phosphorus that can Help You Maintain Good Kidney Health

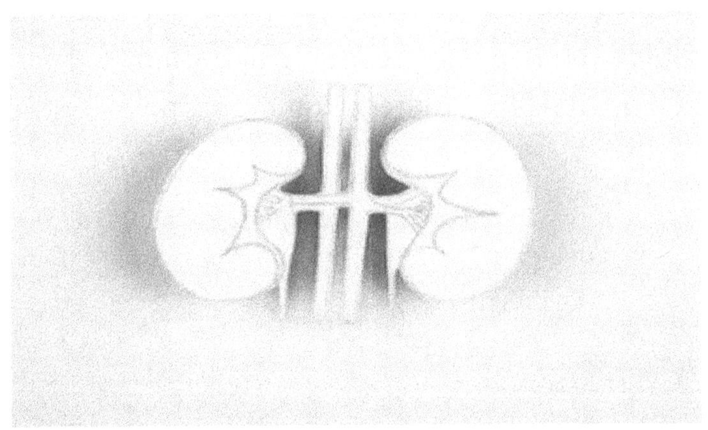

ANDREW POTTER

TABLE OF CONTENTS

CHAPTER ONE
INTRODUCTION
Understanding the Renal Diet

The renal diet is a specific type of food intended to maintain healthy kidney function and control different kidney diseases, such as kidney failure or chronic kidney disease (CKD). In order to lessen the strain on the kidneys, preserve electrolyte balance, and avoid complications related to renal problems, this diet concentrates on controlling the consumption of specific nutrients, namely sodium, potassium, phosphorus, and protein.

Sodium Control: Restricting salt consumption is one of the main components of a renal diet. The kidneys may be further taxed by high blood pressure and fluid retention caused by an excess of salt. When on a renal diet, people usually watch what they eat and cut out on processed and high-sodium meals, preferring to eat fresh, complete foods with flavour from herbs and spices.

Potassium and Phosphorus Management: The body's levels of phosphorus and potassium are controlled by the kidneys. However, these minerals can build up and have negative consequences in kidney-related disorders. Renal diets place a strong emphasis on selecting meals with lower amounts of potassium and phosphorus in order to reduce consumption of these minerals. This entails staying away from specific fruits, veggies, dairy products, and processed meals high in potassium and phosphorus.

Protein Moderation: Although the body needs protein, eating too much of it can strain the kidneys. Diets for the kidneys try to balance the amount of protein consumed in order to avoid waste products from protein breakdown building up. People may be recommended to modify their protein consumption according to their renal function and general health.

In order to customize the diet for their unique needs, people on a renal diet must carefully collaborate with healthcare providers, such as qualified dietitians or nutritionists. Effective management of kidney health requires customized meal planning, frequent evaluation of renal function, and dietary modifications as needed.

Importance of a Kidney-Friendly Diet

A diet that is favourable to the kidneys is crucial for maintaining renal health in general and slowing the development of illnesses connected to the kidneys. The following are important points that highlight how important it is to follow such a food plan:

1. **Optimal Kidney Function:** A diet that is good for the kidneys aids in preserving the body's delicate electrolyte and fluid balance. It helps the kidneys effectively filter waste materials and extra fluid by controlling the intake of minerals including salt, potassium, and phosphorus.

2. **Managing Chronic Kidney Disease (CKD):** Following a kidney-friendly diet becomes essential to the management of chronic kidney disease (CKD) in patients. This dietary strategy helps to minimise problems related to reduced kidney function and to slow down the course of chronic kidney disease (CKD).

3. **Blood Pressure Control:** Blood pressure and kidney health are tightly related. One typical component of kidney-friendly diets is a low-sodium diet, which lowers blood pressure. Lowering salt consumption eases the kidneys' burden and improves cardiovascular health in general.

4. **Preventing Electrolyte Imbalances:** The body's ability to balance electrolytes like potassium and phosphorus depends critically on the kidneys. The requirement to balance these minerals is met by a kidney-friendly diet, which guards against imbalances that can cause problems including muscular weakness, bone problems, and irregular heartbeats.

5. **Delaying Kidney Failure:** A renal-friendly diet can help postpone the need for dialysis or a kidney transplant in situations of severe kidney disease. Reduction of the burden on the kidneys and reduction of toxic material build-up may delay the development of end-stage renal disease.

6. **Enhancing Quality of Life:** Eating a diet that is favourable to the kidneys can help with both treating medical disorders and enhancing general health. It gives people the power to choose food wisely and healthily, promoting their energy and overall well-being.

A renal-friendly diet is essentially a proactive and essential strategy for maintaining kidney function, avoiding difficulties, and encouraging a happier and more satisfying life for those who have or are at risk of kidney-related problems.

CHAPTER TWO
BASICS OF RENAL NUTRITION
Nutrients and their Impact on Kidney Health

Kidney health is greatly impacted by several nutrients. For those with kidney-related disorders, controlling these nutrients through food is essential to maintaining renal function and avoiding complications:

1. **Sodium:** Consuming excessive amounts of salt can raise blood pressure and cause fluid retention, which puts additional strain on the kidneys. Limiting salt lowers the risk of cardiovascular disorders, which are frequently linked to renal problems, and helps control blood pressure.

2. **Potassium:** For the proper functioning of muscles and nerves, potassium levels must be met. However, people with renal problems may be adversely affected by excessive potassium levels. It is vital to keep an eye on potassium

consumption to avoid problems such as irregular heartbeats.

3. **Phosphorus:** The body's phosphorus levels are controlled by the kidneys. Phosphorus levels can rise in response to a reduction in renal function, which can cause heart and bone issues. Limiting meals high in phosphorus aids in controlling blood phosphorus accumulation.

4. **Protein:** Waste products from the degradation of proteins are filtered away by healthy kidneys. Reducing protein consumption helps the kidneys work less hard and accumulate fewer waste products when renal disease is present.

5. **Fluids:** For those with kidney issues, it's critical to keep an eye on their fluid intake to avoid swelling and fluid retention. Limiting the amount of fluid consumed aids in blood pressure control and lessens the kidneys' burden.

6. **Calcium and Vitamin D:** Bone health depends on maintaining adequate quantities of calcium and vitamin D. Bone problems can result from a disruption in the balance of these nutrients in kidney-related ailments. In these

situations, controlling calcium and vitamin D consumption is essential.

Supporting kidney health mostly requires balancing these nutrients through a well-planned diet, frequently under the direction of qualified dietitians or medical specialists. Adjusting consumption in accordance with renal function and personal demands reduces risks and preserves general health.

Portion Control and Meal Planning

The key to maintaining a diet that is kidney-friendly is portion management and careful meal planning. These procedures support the maintenance of general health, the making of educated decisions, and the regulation of nutrient intake in people with kidney-related disorders. This is a summary of their significance:

1. **Managing Sodium and Fluids:**

- Reducing salt consumption is facilitated by portion control, which is important for preserving blood pressure and avoiding fluid retention.
- Controlling portion sizes helps maintain fluid intake, which is important for kidney health, particularly for people with edema.

2. **Balancing Potassium and Phosphorus:**

- Portion control can help prevent imbalances that might be dangerous for those with impaired kidney function by controlling the amount of foods high in potassium and phosphorus that are consumed.
- People can enjoy a range of foods while adhering to suggested intake levels for these minerals by carefully arranging their meals.

3. **Moderating Protein Intake:**

- Planning meals enables you to distribute protein over the course of the day, which lessens the strain on your kidneys.
- A healthy diet that limits portions guarantees that people get enough protein without going overboard and taxing their kidneys.

4. **Optimizing Nutrient Intake:**
   - Meal preparation in advance makes it easier to eat a balanced diet that contains the elements your body needs to function properly.
   - Portion control ensures people get the nutrients they need without taxing their kidneys by preventing overconsumption.

5. **Customizing to Individual Needs:**
   - A customized approach to meal planning is made possible by customizing portion sizes to meet individual needs, taking into account variables such as age, weight, and kidney function.
   - Customization guarantees that dietary guidelines correspond with particular health objectives and limitations.

6. **Promoting Consistency:**
   - Meal planning and portion management are important aspects of regular dietary practises, which are especially important for those with chronic renal disease.
   - Long-term adherence to dietary recommendations is supported by consistency, which improves kidney health outcomes.

People may maintain renal health and yet enjoy a diverse and enjoyable diet by combining meal planning with quantity management. Seeking advice from dietitians or medical specialists can offer tailored recommendations for optimising these practises according to specific health requirements.

Foods to Limit or Avoid

In order to promote kidney health, a kidney-friendly diet usually involves limiting or avoiding specific foods. The following lists and illustrations of often prohibited foods are:

1. **High-Sodium Foods:**
    - Processed meats (like bacon, deli meats)
    - Canned soups and broths
    - Pickled and canned vegetables
    - Fast foods and restaurant meals high in sodium
2. **High-Potassium Foods:**
    - Bananas
    - Oranges and orange juice
    - Potatoes (including sweet potatoes)
    - Tomatoes and tomato products (sauce, paste)
3. **High-Phosphorus Foods:**
    - Dairy products (milk, cheese, yogurt)
    - Nuts and seeds (almonds, peanuts)
    - Colas and dark sodas
    - Whole grains and bran cereals

4. **High-Protein Foods (in excessive amounts):**
    - Red meat (beef, lamb)
    - Poultry (chicken, turkey)

- Fish and shellfish
- Eggs (especially yolks)

5. **Processed Foods and Additives:**
   - Convenience foods (packaged snacks, frozen meals)
   - High-phosphorus additives (phosphoric acid, sodium phosphate)
   - Artificial sweeteners containing phosphorus (aspartame)

6. **Certain Beverages:**
   - Alcohol in excess
   - Sugary drinks and high-phosphorus beverages
   - Energy drinks and certain herbal teas (like star anise tea)

7. **Excessive Fluids:**
   - Limiting fluids is essential for those who need to manage fluid retention or have fluid-related issues such as edema.

Recall that dietary limits for each person may differ depending on their unique kidney health demands, so it's important to speak with a medical expert or a qualified dietitian to create a customised diet plan. Even with meals that are thought to be healthy in moderation for those with renal problems, portion management and moderation are crucial.

CHAPTER THREE
BUILDING A KIDNEY-FRIENDLY PLATE

Guidelines for Balanced Meals

Making well-balanced meals is crucial for those who adhere to a diet low in kidney stones. To guarantee a comprehensive and wholesome approach to meal planning, follow these guidelines:

1. **Incorporate a Variety of Foods:** To guarantee a wide range of nutrients, incorporate a variety of fruits, vegetables, whole grains, lean meats, and healthy fats.

2. **Pay Attention to Portion Sizes:** Regulate portion sizes to control your consumption of phosphorus, potassium, and salt. This promotes overall renal health and helps avoid overtaxing the kidneys.

3. **Select Lean Proteins:** Go for plant-based proteins like beans and tofu as well as lean protein sources like fish, chicken, and eggs. This aids in controlling protein consumption without putting undue load on the kidneys.

4. **Prioritize Colorful Vegetables:** Add a range of vibrant veggies as they are a good source of vitamins and minerals. But be aware of high-potassium foods and adjust portion sizes accordingly.

5. **Limit Processed meals:** Try consuming as little as possible of packaged and processed meals, which frequently have high salt content and potentially harmful ingredients.

6. **Pick Whole Grains:** Refined grains should be avoided in favor of whole grains such brown rice, quinoa, and whole wheat. They supply minerals and fiber without adding to the phosphorus excess.

7. **Monitor Fluid Intake:** Pay attention to how much fluid you consume, particularly if you are told to restrict it. Drink fluids in moderation throughout the day to prevent the kidneys from being overworked at once.

8. **Use Healthy Fats:** Incorporate moderate amounts of foods high in healthful fats, such as almonds, avocados, and olive oil. They improve general health without having a negative impact on renal function.

9. **Be Aware of Dairy:** Select lower-phosphorus dairy choices, such as modest quantities of dairy products or milk replacements, if you're told to restrict phosphorus. Think about substitutes such as rice or almond milk.

10. **Minimize Salt and Added Sugars:** Reduce the amount of food that has salt and added sugars. Instead of using too much salt for flavor, utilize herbs and spices as natural sweeteners.

11. **Consult a Nutritionist:** To develop a customized meal plan that takes into account dietary limitations and specific health concerns, collaborate with a trained nutritionist.

By following these guidelines, individuals can enjoy flavorful and satisfying meals while promoting kidney health and overall well-being. Regular monitoring and adjustments, guided by healthcare professionals, ensure a sustainable and effective approach to managing kidney-related conditions.

Choosing the Right Proteins, Carbohydrates, and Fats

Choosing the Right Proteins:

1. **Lean Protein Sources:** Choose lean proteins like fish, skinless chicken, and lean beef portions. These options supply necessary amino acids without having too much saturated fat.

2. **Plant-Based Proteins:** Add in sources of plant-based protein such as edamame, lentils, beans, and tofu. These choices can be beneficial substitutes for people managing renal health since they often contain less phosphorus.

3. **Egg Whites:** As an excellent source of protein that has less phosphorus than whole eggs, think about including egg whites.

4. **Dairy Substitutes:** If phosphorus is an issue for you, consider dairy substitutes like rice or almond milk, which are frequently lower in phosphorus.

Choosing the Right Carbohydrates:

1. **Whole Grains:** Place a focus on whole grains such as whole wheat bread, quinoa, and brown rice. These offer fiber and necessary minerals without adding an excessive amount of phosphorus.

2. **Limit Refined Carbohydrates:** Cut less on foods high in sugar, such as white bread and sugar-filled snacks. Choose complex carbs to promote general well-being.

3. **Regulated Portion Sizes:** Keep an eye on portion sizes to control your consumption of carbohydrates. For those who need to keep an eye on their phosphorus levels, this is especially crucial.

4. **Fruits and Vegetables:** Choose fruits and vegetables that are lower in potassium if necessary, but include a range of them in moderation. Manage portion sizes to maintain a balanced diet.

Choosing the Right Fats:

1. **Healthy Oils:** When cooking, choose heart-healthy oils like canola or olive oil. They supply monounsaturated fats without adding to the phosphorus problems.

2. **Nuts and Seeds in Moderation:** As a source of good fats, take pleasure in nuts and seeds in moderation. Think about lower-phosphorus foods such as almonds.

3. **Avocados**: As a good source of monounsaturated fats, including avocados in moderation. To control your consumption of phosphorus, pay attention to portion sizes.

4. **Fatty Fish:** To get your omega-3 fatty acids, try including fatty fish like mackerel and salmon. They support heart health without having a major effect on phosphorus levels.

Recall that every person has different nutritional requirements, therefore seeking the advice of a certified dietitian or other healthcare provider is essential for tailored advice. They can help tailor dietary choices based on specific health conditions and ensure a well-balanced and kidney-friendly approach to nutrition.

CHAPTER FOUR
GROCERY SHOPPING FOR RENAL HEALTH

Essential Ingredients

1. **Fresh Vegetables:** Select a range of vibrant, low-potassium veggies, such as bell peppers, cauliflower, and broccoli. These supply vital minerals and vitamins.

2. **Berries:** Choose blueberries, raspberries, and strawberries among other berries. When compared to certain other fruits, they have less potassium.

3. **Lean Proteins:** Choose lean protein sources, such as fish, eggs, skinless chicken, and plant-based proteins like tofu and beans. They supply the necessary amino acids without having too much phosphorus.

4. **Entire Grains:** Use entire grains such as whole wheat bread, quinoa, and brown rice. These provide fiber and essential nutrients without adding an excessive amount of phosphorus.

5. **Olive Oil:** When cooking, use heart-healthy oils like olive oil. It enhances flavor without adding to phosphorus issues.

6. **Low-Phosphorus Dairy Alternatives:** If you must restrict your intake of phosphorus from conventional dairy sources, consider dairy substitutes like rice or almond milk.

7. **Egg Whites:** Since egg whites have less phosphorus than whole eggs, you may choose to use them as a source of protein.

8. **Herbs and Spices:** Instead of using too much salt, add flavor with herbs and spices like turmeric, thyme, and basil.

9. **Nuts and Seeds in Moderation:** Choose lower-phosphorus choices, such as almonds, and enjoy nuts and seeds in moderation.

10. **Fruits in Moderation:** To limit potassium consumption, eat fruits like apples, cherries, and grapes in portion-controlled amounts.

11. **Garlic and Onions:** Add flavor to your food without raising any issues with phosphorus or potassium.

12. **Cauliflower Rice:** To cut back on phosphorus intake, swap out ordinary rice for cauliflower rice.

13. **Low-Phosphorus Pasta:** Choose low-phosphorus pastas that are manufactured using rice or maize flour as an alternative.

14. **Fresh Herbs:** To enhance flavor, add fresh herbs like mint, cilantro, and parsley.

15. Fish with Omega-3 Fatty Acids: For heart-healthy omega-3 fatty acids, including fatty fish like mackerel and salmon.

Always remember to adjust ingredient selections to suit specific dietary needs, and seek the guidance of dietitians or medical specialists for individualized nutritional management of kidney health.

Reading Food Labels

1. **Serving Size:** To begin with, make sure the serving size fits your dietary requirements by verifying it. This serving size serves as the basis for all nutritional information on the label.

2. **Sodium Content:** Seek for low-sodium items; try to find servings that contain no more than 140 mg of sodium. Terms such as "monosodium glutamate" and "sodium chloride" should be used with caution.

3. **Potassium and Phosphorus Levels:** Check the levels of these minerals, particularly if you need to restrict them. Select lower-level foods or modify portion amounts accordingly.

4. **Protein Content:** Pay attention to your protein intake, particularly if you're following a diet low in protein. Select meals with moderate protein content and think about modifying serving sizes according to your individual requirements.

5. **Phosphorus Additives:** Look for additions like sodium phosphate or phosphoric acid that contain phosphorus. Products with a lot of these ingredients should be limited.

6. **Hidden Sodium Sources:** Recognise the sources of hidden sodium that might add to your daily consumption, such as baking soda, baking powder, and sodium benzoate.

7. **Hidden Sources of Phosphorus:** Keep an eye out for additions like phosphoric acid and sodium hexametaphosphate that may include hidden sources of phosphorus.

8. **Added Sugars:** Select goods with low sugar content to reduce added sugar intake. Use caution when referring to sugar by other terms, such as sucrose or high-fructose corn syrup.

9. **Trans Fats and Saturated Fats:** Limit saturated fats and steer clear of items in trans fats. Choose foods high in monounsaturated and polyunsaturated fats, which are healthier fat sources.

10. **Ingredient List:** Examine the ingredient list to find any unlisted preservatives and additions. Learn about words that might refer to additives containing phosphorus.

11. **Dairy Substitutes:** Select dairy substitutes that are fortified with calcium and vitamin D. Make sure the phosphorus content is minimal.

12. **Fresh and Whole Foods:** Give fresh and whole foods first priority whenever you can. They offer more control over nutritional intake and have less additives by nature.

By educating yourself on food labels, you may adjust your diet to suit your needs for kidney health. When in doubt, consult with a registered dietitian for personalized guidance based on your specific dietary restrictions and health requirements.

CHAPTER FIVE
ESSENTIAL NUTRIENTS

Sodium Management

Effective Sodium Management for Kidney Health:

1. **Read Food Labels:** Examine food labels carefully to determine the salt amount. Choose items with the labels "low sodium" or "sodium-free," and keep an eye out for sodium that may be concealed in additives.

2. **Select Fresh, Whole Foods:** Give fresh produce, raw meats, and fruits first priority. These have naturally lower salt content than packaged and processed meals.

3. **Cook at Home:** Make meals using fresh ingredients at your house. This facilitates more control over salt intake and encourages a more nutritious diet.

4. **Limit Processed Foods:** Because processed and packaged foods frequently have high salt content, limit your consumption of these items. Pick whole, raw options wherever you can.

5. **Use Herbs and Spices:** Instead of using salt, add flavor using herbs, spices, and other seasonings. Experiment with garlic, onion, lemon, and various herbs to add depth without increasing sodium.

6. **Be Wary of Condiments:** Verify the amount of salt in salad dressings, ketchup, and soy sauce, among other condiments. To reduce salt levels, use low-sodium options or prepare your own at home.

7. **Rinse Canned Foods:** Before eating any canned goods, such as beans or veggies, give them a quick wash under running water. This lowers the amount of sodium.

8. **Restrict the Use of High-Sodium items:** Restrict the use of high-sodium items including sauces, bottled broths, and bouillon cubes. Investigate low-sodium substitutes or prepare homemade broths.

9. **Select Low-Sodium Snacks:** Go for low-sodium snack alternatives including fresh fruit and vegetables, air-popped popcorn, or unsalted almonds.

10. **Limit Processed Meats:** Because they frequently have high salt content, limit your intake of processed meats like bacon, sausage and deli meats. Instead, go for lean, fresh protein sources.

11. **Monitor Restaurant Choices:** To limit your salt consumption when dining out, ask for sauces and dressings on the side or ask for lower-sodium choices.

12. **Stay Hydrated:** Maintaining enough fluid balance will assist control the body's salt levels, so make sure you're getting plenty of it.

13. **Gradual Reduction:** Aim for a gradual reduction if your diet has been higher in salt. Your taste receptors might adapt as a result over time.

Maintaining ideal blood pressure and lessening the burden on the kidneys may be achieved by implementing these practices, which are essential for sodium control and renal health. Always seek the advice of licensed dietitians or medical specialists for individualized recommendations based on your unique health requirements.

Potassium Regulation

Strategies for Potassium Regulation in a Kidney-Friendly Diet:

1. **Monitor Potassium Levels:** As directed by medical specialists, periodically monitor potassium levels through blood tests to inform dietary modifications.

2. **Select Low-Potassium Fruits and Vegetables:** Go for fruits and veggies like apples, berries, and green beans that are lower in potassium. Pay attention to serving sizes.

3. **Limit High-Potassium Foods:** Cut back on the amount of foods high in potassium, such as oranges, potatoes, tomatoes, bananas, and orange juice. To control potassium consumption, watch portion sizes.

4. **Soak and Boil Potatoes:** To extract part of the potassium, soak potatoes in water before boiling. Throw away the water that was used to soak.

5. **Explore Lower-Potassium Grains:** Choose lower-potassium grains like white rice and couscous over higher-potassium ones like quinoa and brown rice.

6. **Pick Lean Proteins:** Lean protein choices with reduced potassium content include fish, eggs, and chicken. Pay attention to serving sizes.

7. **Reduce Dairy Intake:** If potassium restriction is recommended, reduce dairy consumption and opt for lower-potassium substitutes such as rice or almond milk.

8. **Rinse Canned Foods:** Before eating, rinse canned beans, vegetables, and legumes to lower their potassium level.

9. **Steer Clear of High-Potassium Additives:** KCL is a common alternative for salt; be wary of such additions. Look for these ingredients on food labels.

10. **Cooking Techniques Matter:** Instead of baking or roasting, which may concentrate potassium, choose cooking procedures like boiling that lower potassium levels.

11. **Limit High-Potassium Snacks:** Steer clear of high-potassium snacks like dried fruits and choose instead for low-potassium choices like unsalted almonds.

12. **Stay Hydrated:** Keeping the body properly hydrated is important for controlling potassium levels.

13. **Consult a Dietitian:** For individualized advice on controlling potassium levels based on your unique medical circumstances, work with a trained dietitian.

For kidney health, potassium consumption must be balanced. These tips can help people eat a wide range of foods and keep their potassium levels at their ideal levels. Maintaining a customized approach to potassium management based on specific health situations is ensured by regular consultation with healthcare providers.

Phosphorus Control

Strategies for Phosphorus Control in a Kidney-Friendly Diet:

1. **Monitor Phosphorus Levels:** Follow doctor's recommendations and routinely check blood levels for phosphorus to inform dietary changes.

2. **Select Low-Phosphorus Proteins:** Go for fish, poultry, and chicken as examples of proteins that are lower in phosphorus. Limit your consumption of high-phosphorus proteins, such as shellfish and organ meats.

3. **Control Dairy Consumption:** Because dairy items are high in phosphorus, limit your intake of dairy products. Opt for lower-phosphorus substitutes such as rice or almond milk.

4. **Limit Processed Foods:** Because processed and packaged foods sometimes have additives with a high phosphorus concentration, consume them as little as possible. Whenever possible, go for complete, fresh meals.

5. **Control Portion Sizes:** Pay attention to portion sizes to prevent consuming too much phosphorus, particularly from foods high in phosphorus such as whole grains, nuts, and seeds.

6. **Knowledge of Phosphorus Additives:** Look for additives such as sodium phosphate and phosphoric acid on food labels that contain phosphorus. Products with a lot of these ingredients should be limited.

7. **Methods for Soaking and Draining:** Before cooking, soak beans and legumes. To lower the phosphorus level in canned beans and legumes, drain and rinse them.

8. **Restrict Dark Cola Use:** Steer clear of dark colas since they contain phosphoric acid, which raises the levels of phosphorus in the body. Choose water or clear drinks instead.

9. **Opt for White Breads:** Since white bread usually contains less phosphorus than whole wheat or whole grain alternatives, choose it instead.

10. **Cooking Methods Matter:** Instead of roasting or other cooking techniques that might concentrate phosphorus, use techniques like boiling that lower the amount of phosphorus in food.

11. **Limit Supplements containing Phosphorus:** If supplements are recommended, follow doctor's instructions. Steer clear of over-the-counter supplements unless advised.

12. **Drink plenty of water:** Drink enough water, since this can assist control the body's phosphorus levels.

13. **Work closely with a Dietitian:** For individualized advice on controlling phosphorus levels based on your unique health needs, collaborate with a qualified dietitian.

For kidney health, phosphorus consumption must be balanced. These tips can help people keep their phosphorus levels at their ideal levels while still eating a varied and nourishing diet. Maintaining a customized strategy to phosphorus management based on individual health factors is ensured by regular consultation with healthcare providers.

CHAPTER SIX
COOKING TECHNIQUES FOR RENAL DIETS

Low-Sodium Cooking

Tips for Low-Sodium Cooking in a Kidney-Friendly Diet:

1. **Fresh Herbs and Spices:** Use flavorings such as basil, thyme, oregano, and rosemary that are fresh to avoid using salt.

2. **Citrus Zest and Juices:** Add a taste explosion to meals by using the zest and juice of citrus fruits like oranges, lemons, and limes.

3. **Vinegars:** To give your food some tang, try experimenting with various vinegars, including apple cider or balsamic.

4. **Garlic and Onions:** Use fresh or powdered garlic and onions to give your meals a savory touch.

5. **Homemade Seasonings:** For a customized flavor profile, make your own seasoning mixes with a range of herbs, spices, and aromatics.

6. **Low-Sodium Broths:** For the foundation of soups, stews, and sauces, use low-sodium or sodium-free broths and bouillons.

7. **Limit Use of Salt Substitutes:** Use caution and seek medical advice before substituting salt; some may include potassium or other minerals that should be watched.

8. **Grilling and Roasting:** Without using a lot of salt, enhance the natural flavors of meats and vegetables by using grilling and roasting techniques.

9. **Fresh components:** To better limit salt levels, give preference to entire, fresh components over processed or pre-packaged foods.

10. **Rinse Canned Foods:** Before using canned beans, veggies, and legumes in recipes, carefully rinse them under water to lower their salt level.

11. **Reduce or Avoid High-Sodium Condiments:** Use caution while consuming high-sodium condiments such as Worcestershire sauce, soy sauce, and certain dressings. Choose low-sodium substitutes or use them in moderation.

12. **Herb-infused Oils:** To enhance the flavor of olive oil, mix with herbs such as thyme or rosemary to create herb-infused oils.

13. **Teach Your Palate:** Gradually cut down on the salt in your dishes so that, over time, your palate can get used to reduced sodium levels.

14. **Homemade Marinades:** Instead of choosing high-sodium choices, flavor meats using homemade marinades prepared with vinegar, citrus liquids, and herbs.

15. **Label Awareness:** When buying pre-packaged foods, carefully read the labels and select those that are labeled as sodium-free or low-sodium.

Cooking with low salt not only helps kidney health but also fosters a rich and varied culinary experience. Try a variety of herbs, spices, and cooking methods to find delectable substitutes for foods heavy in salt.

Flavoring with Herbs and Spices

Enhancing Flavor with Herbs and Spices in a Kidney-Friendly Diet:

1. **Basil:** Basil, either fresh or dried, offers a flavor that is sweet and somewhat spicy. Add it to salads, sauces, and pasta meals.
2. **Thyme:** Thyme has a faintly citrusy and earthy taste. It goes well with soups, roasted veggies, and chicken.
3. **Rosemary:** When added to roasted meats, potatoes, and bread, rosemary imparts a peppery and piney flavor.
4. **Oregano:** A versatile herb that tastes great in pizza, pasta, and salads, oregano may be used either fresh or dried.

5. **Cilantro:** Cilantro adds a zesty, fresh flavor to guacamole, salsas, and a variety of ethnic dishes.

6. **Parsley:** Parsley is a multipurpose plant with a mild, somewhat peppery flavor. Use it as a garnish and in salads and soups.

7. **Chives:** With its subtle onion flavor, chives make a delicious salad, omelet, or baked potato topping.

8. **Dill:** Dill has a unique flavor with notes of anise and lemon. It goes nicely with fish, potatoes, and recipes that contain yogurt.

9. **Mint:** Mint offers a pleasant and refreshing touch. Add it to drinks, salads, or desserts as a garnish.

10. **Coriander:** This herb has warm, lemony undertones when used in both its seeds and fresh leaves (cilantro). Utilize them in spice mixes, marinades, and curries.

11. **Garlic:** Roasted or fresh garlic adds flavor to savory foods. It may be used in nearly any type of cooking.

12. **Ginger:** Ginger gives savory and sweet foods a sense of depth and warmth. Add it to soups, marinades, and stir-fries.

13. **Turmeric:** The earthy, somewhat bitter, and warm flavor of turmeric is imparted. It's a crucial component of many curry recipes and spice combinations.

14. **Paprika:** There are several varieties of paprika, and each has a distinct flavor. It gives stews, soups, and roasted vegetables more color and depth.

15. **Cumin:** Often used in Middle Eastern, Indian, and Mexican cooking, cumin has a toasty, nutty flavor. It goes well with meats, beans, and rice dishes.

You may follow a kidney-friendly diet and create countless flavor combinations by experimenting with these herbs and spices. Enhancing the flavor of meats, veggies, or grains may be accomplished with the appropriate mix, which can elevate an ordinary dish to a gourmet experience.

CHAPTER SEVEN
BREAKFAST DELIGHTS
Kidney-Friendly Smoothies

1. **Berry Blast:**
   - **Ingredients:** Mixed berries (strawberries, blueberries, raspberries), low-potassium yogurt or almond milk, ice.
   - **Optional:** Add a touch of honey or a squeeze of lemon for extra flavor.
2. **Cucumber Mint Cooler:**
   - **Ingredients:** Cucumber, fresh mint leaves, low-potassium yogurt, ice.
   - **Optional:** A splash of lime juice for a refreshing twist.
3. **Pineapple Paradise:**
   - **Ingredients:** Pineapple chunks, banana (in moderation), coconut water, ice.
   - **Optional:** A sprinkle of chia seeds for added texture.

4. **Citrus Delight:**
   - **Ingredients:** Oranges, kiwi, low-potassium yogurt or almond milk, ice.
   - **Optional:** A dash of vanilla extract for a subtle sweetness.

5. **Avocado Banana Bliss:**
   - **Ingredients:** Avocado, banana (in moderation), low-potassium yogurt or almond milk, ice.
   - **Optional:** A drizzle of agave syrup for extra sweetness.

6. **Melon Medley:**
   - **Ingredients:** Cantaloupe or honeydew melon, cucumber, low-potassium yogurt or coconut water, ice.
   - **Optional:** Fresh basil leaves for a hint of herbal flavor.

7. **Mango Tango:**
   - **Ingredients:** Mango chunks, pineapple, low-potassium yogurt or almond milk, ice.
   - **Optional:** A pinch of turmeric for added color and potential anti-inflammatory benefits.

8. **Green Goddess:**
   - **Ingredients:** Spinach, kale, green apple, low-potassium yogurt or coconut water, ice.
   - **Optional:** A squeeze of lemon or lime juice for brightness.
9. **Cherry Almond Dream:**
   - **Ingredients:** Cherries, almond milk, a handful of spinach, ice.
   - **Optional:** A sprinkle of ground flaxseeds for an omega-3 boost.
10. **Peachy Keen:**
   - **Ingredients:** Peaches, banana (in moderation), low-potassium yogurt or almond milk, ice.
   - **Optional:** A dash of cinnamon for warmth.

Remember to tailor these recipes based on your specific dietary needs and restrictions. Adjusting portion sizes and choosing low-potassium alternatives ensures that these smoothies align with a kidney-friendly diet. If in doubt, consult with a healthcare professional or a registered dietitian for personalized advice.

Low-Phosphorus Breakfast Options

1. **Egg White Omelette:** Fill an omelette with colorful vegetables like bell peppers, spinach, and tomatoes. Use egg whites for a protein-packed, low-phosphorus option.

2. **Greek Yogurt Parfait:** Choose low-phosphorus Greek yogurt and layer it with fresh berries, a sprinkle of nuts (in moderation), and a drizzle of honey for sweetness.

3. **Oatmeal with Berries:** Prepare oatmeal with water or a low-phosphorus milk substitute. Top it with fresh berries and a dash of cinnamon for flavor.

4. **Smoothie Bowl:** Create a smoothie bowl using low-potassium fruits like berries and banana (in moderation). Add a dollop of low-phosphorus yogurt and sprinkle with seeds or nuts (in moderation).

5. **Rice Cake with Avocado:** Top a rice cake with sliced avocado and a sprinkle of sesame seeds for a satisfying and low-phosphorus breakfast.

6. **Homemade Muffins:** Bake low-phosphorus muffins using ingredients like white flour, applesauce, and egg whites. Customize with berries or a touch of vanilla for flavor.

7. **Cottage Cheese and Fruit Bowl:** Choose a low-phosphorus cottage cheese and pair it with fresh, low-potassium fruits like peaches or melon for a simple and tasty breakfast.

8. **Vegetable and Tofu Scramble:** Saute tofu with low-phosphorus vegetables like zucchini, bell peppers, and spinach for a nutrient-rich and kidney-friendly scramble.

9. **Quinoa Breakfast Bowl:** Cook quinoa with water or a low-phosphorus broth and top it with diced apples, a sprinkle of cinnamon, and a handful of almonds (in moderation).

10. **Pancakes with Berries:** Prepare low-phosphorus pancakes using a mix of white flour and egg whites. Top with fresh berries and a dollop of low-phosphorus whipped cream.

11. **Cereal with Low-Phosphorus Milk:** Choose a low-phosphorus cereal and pair it with a milk substitute like almond milk or rice milk for a quick and easy breakfast.

12. **Fruit Salad:** Create a refreshing fruit salad using low-potassium fruits like strawberries, blueberries, and pineapple. Add a squeeze of lime juice for extra flavor.

Always consider your individual dietary needs and consult with a healthcare professional or registered dietitian for personalized guidance on low-phosphorus breakfast options tailored to your specific kidney health requirements.

Egg substitutes and Renal-Friendly Omelets

For those looking to reduce egg consumption or following a renal-friendly diet, several egg substitutes can be used to create omelets with similar texture and flavor. Here are some options:

1. **Egg Whites:** Use only the egg whites, as they are lower in phosphorus compared to the yolks. Egg whites can still provide the fluffiness and protein content needed for an omelet.

2. **Tofu:** Silken tofu, when blended, can mimic the texture of scrambled eggs. Add your favorite vegetables and seasonings for a tasty tofu omelet.

3. **Chickpea Flour (Besan):** Make a batter using chickpea flour, water, and seasonings. Cook it into a pancake-like consistency and fold it around sautéed vegetables for a chickpea flour omelet.

4. **Legume Flour (Lentil or Pea Flour):** Similarly to chickpea flour, you can use lentil or pea flour mixed with water to create a batter for a protein-rich omelet.

5. **Egg Replacer Powders:** Commercial egg replacer powders, made from potato starch, tapioca flour, and leavening agents, can be used to create an egg-like texture in omelets.

Renal-Friendly Omelet Recipe:

Ingredients:
- 3/4 cup egg whites
- 1/4 cup silken tofu, blended
- 1/2 cup diced low-potassium vegetables (e.g., bell peppers, spinach, mushrooms)
- 1 tablespoon olive oil
- Salt and pepper to taste

Instructions:

1. **Prepare Vegetables:** Sauté diced vegetables in olive oil until they are tender. Set aside.

2. **Blend Tofu:** In a blender, blend silken tofu until smooth.

3. **Mix Ingredients:** In a bowl, mix egg whites, blended tofu, and sautéed vegetables. Add salt and pepper to taste.

4. **Cook Omelet:** Heat a non-stick pan over medium heat. Pour the mixture into the pan and cook until the edges are set. Flip or fold the omelet to cook evenly.

5. **Serve:** Slide the omelet onto a plate and serve hot.

Remember to customize the recipe based on your specific dietary needs and consult with a healthcare professional or a registered dietitian for personalized guidance on renal-friendly meal options.

CHAPTER EIGHT
SATISFYING LUNCH IDEAS
Protein-Packed Main Dishes

1. **Grilled Chicken Breast:** Season with herbs and spices, then grill or bake for a lean and protein-rich option.

2. **Baked Fish Fillets:** Choose white fish like cod or tilapia and bake with lemon, herbs, and a drizzle of olive oil.

3. **Tofu and Vegetable Stir-Fry:** Stir-fry tofu with low-potassium vegetables in a kidney-friendly sauce made with low-sodium soy sauce, ginger, and garlic.

4. **Egg White Frittata:** Whisk egg whites and cook with vegetables like spinach, tomatoes, and mushrooms for a protein-packed frittata.

5. **Salmon with Herbed Quinoa:** Grill or bake salmon and serve it with a side of herbed quinoa for a complete and nutritious meal.

6. **Lentil and Vegetable Curry:** Make a kidney-friendly curry with lentils, low-potassium vegetables, and a mild blend of spices.

7. **Turkey and Vegetable Skewers:** Skewer lean turkey pieces with low-potassium vegetables, then grill or bake for a tasty and protein-packed dish.

8. **Chickpea Salad:** Toss chickpeas with diced cucumbers, tomatoes, and herbs. Drizzle with olive oil and lemon juice for a refreshing salad.

9. **Quinoa and Black Bean Bowl:** Combine quinoa with black beans, corn, and diced tomatoes. Season with cumin, coriander, and lime for a flavorful bowl.

10. **Baked Chicken Thighs with Herbs:** Bake chicken thighs with a mix of kidney-friendly herbs like thyme, rosemary, and parsley for a flavorful dish.

11. **Vegetarian Stuffed Bell Peppers:** Fill bell peppers with a mixture of quinoa, black beans, corn, and tomatoes. Bake until peppers are tender.

12. **Greek Salad with Grilled Chicken:** Top a Greek salad with grilled chicken, feta cheese, olives, and a kidney-friendly dressing.

13. **Shrimp and Broccoli Stir-Fry:** Stir-fry shrimp with broccoli, bell peppers, and snap peas in a low-sodium soy sauce for a quick and protein-packed meal.

14. **Baked Cod with Tomato Salsa:** Bake cod fillets and top with a fresh tomato salsa made with cilantro, lime, and diced tomatoes.

15. **Quinoa and Chicken Bowl:** Combine quinoa with grilled chicken, roasted vegetables, and a squeeze of lemon for a satisfying bowl.

Always consider individual dietary needs, including potassium and phosphorus restrictions, and consult with a healthcare professional or registered dietitian for personalized guidance on renal-friendly meal options.

Vegetarian and Plant-Based Options

1. **Lentil Soup:** Make a hearty lentil soup with low-potassium vegetables and kidney-friendly herbs and spices.

2. **Quinoa Salad:** Create a refreshing quinoa salad with cucumber, cherry tomatoes, and a lemon vinaigrette.

3. **Stuffed Portobello Mushrooms:** Fill portobello mushrooms with a mixture of kidney-friendly grains, vegetables, and herbs, then bake until tender.

4. **Chickpea and Spinach Curry:** Cook chickpeas and spinach in a kidney-friendly curry sauce made with low-sodium tomatoes, ginger, and garlic.

5. **Sweet Potato and Black Bean Tacos:** Fill whole-grain tortillas with roasted sweet potatoes, black beans, and a cilantro-lime sauce.

6. **Eggplant and Tomato Bake:** Layer sliced eggplant and tomatoes in a baking dish, season with herbs, and bake for a flavorful dish.

7. **Vegetarian Stir-Fry:** Stir-fry a variety of low-potassium vegetables like broccoli, bell peppers, and snap peas with tofu or tempeh.

8. **Zucchini Noodles with Pesto:** Replace traditional pasta with zucchini noodles and top with a kidney-friendly pesto sauce.

9. **Spinach and Feta Stuffed Bell Peppers:** Stuff bell peppers with a mixture of spinach, feta cheese, and kidney-friendly herbs. Bake until peppers are tender.

10. **Cauliflower and Chickpea Curry:** Make a curry using cauliflower and chickpeas with kidney-friendly spices like turmeric and cumin.

11. **Black Bean and Vegetable Quesadillas:** Fill whole-grain tortillas with black beans, sautéed vegetables, and a sprinkle of kidney-friendly cheese.

12. **Mushroom and Spinach Risotto:** Prepare a creamy mushroom and spinach risotto using arborio rice and low-sodium vegetable broth.

13. **Grilled Tofu Skewers:** Marinate tofu cubes in a kidney-friendly sauce and grill them on skewers with colorful vegetables.

14. **Cabbage and White Bean Soup:** Cook cabbage and white beans in a flavorful broth with kidney-friendly seasonings.

15. **Mango and Avocado Salad:** Toss together diced mango, avocado, and mixed greens. Dress with a kidney-friendly vinaigrette.

Remember to adapt these recipes based on individual dietary needs and restrictions. Consulting with a healthcare professional or a registered dietitian is essential for personalized guidance on renal-friendly vegetarian and plant-based meal options.

Soups and Stew for Nutrient-Rich meal

1. **Vegetable and Lentil Soup:** Combine a variety of low-potassium vegetables with lentils in a flavorful broth seasoned with kidney-friendly herbs.

2. **Chicken and Vegetable Stew:** Make a hearty stew with lean chicken, carrots, celery, and potatoes in a low-sodium chicken broth.

3. **Minestrone Soup:** Create a nutrient-packed minestrone soup with kidney-friendly vegetables, beans, and whole-grain pasta.

4. **Turmeric and Ginger Lentil Stew:** Cook lentils with turmeric, ginger, and a mix of kidney-friendly vegetables for a comforting and anti-inflammatory stew.

5. **Tomato and Basil Quinoa Soup:** Blend tomatoes and basil into a broth, then add quinoa and kidney-friendly vegetables for a nourishing soup.

6. **Barley and Mushroom Soup:** Simmer barley with mushrooms, carrots, and onions in a low-sodium vegetable broth for a hearty and nutrient-rich soup.

7. **Chickpea and Spinach Stew:** Combine chickpeas, spinach, and tomatoes in a kidney-friendly broth with garlic and cumin for a flavorful stew.

8. **Chicken and Rice Soup:** Prepare a classic chicken and rice soup using low-sodium chicken broth, diced chicken, and kidney-friendly vegetables.

9. **Sweet Potato and Black Bean Chili:** Make a nutrient-rich chili using sweet potatoes, black beans, tomatoes, and kidney-friendly spices like cumin and chili powder.

10. **Butternut Squash and Apple Soup:** Blend roasted butternut squash and apples into a creamy soup, seasoned with kidney-friendly herbs.

11. **Red Lentil and Vegetable Curry Soup:** Cook red lentils with kidney-friendly vegetables in a curry-spiced broth for a flavorful and nutrient-packed soup.

12. **Spinach and White Bean Stew:** Simmer white beans with spinach, tomatoes, and herbs in a low-sodium vegetable broth for a nourishing stew.

13. **Cabbage and Potato Soup:** Combine cabbage, potatoes, and carrots in a kidney-friendly broth for a hearty and nutrient-rich soup.

14. **Quinoa and Black Bean Stew:** Cook quinoa and black beans with kidney-friendly vegetables in a flavorful stew with cumin and coriander.

15. **Mushroom and Barley Soup:** Create a comforting mushroom and barley soup with kidney-friendly herbs like thyme and rosemary.

These soups and stews offer a balance of nutrients while adhering to kidney-friendly guidelines. Adjust recipes based on individual dietary needs, and consult with healthcare professionals or registered dietitians for personalized guidance on renal-friendly meal options.

Sandwiches with Low-Sodium Options

1. **Turkey and Avocado Wrap:** Fill a whole-grain wrap with sliced turkey, avocado, lettuce, and tomato. Use a kidney-friendly dressing or mustard for flavor.

2. **Grilled Chicken and Vegetable Panini:** Grill chicken breast with low-potassium vegetables like bell peppers and zucchini. Place them between whole-grain bread and press for a delicious panini.

3. **Egg Salad Lettuce Wraps:** Make a low-sodium egg salad with Greek yogurt, mustard, and herbs. Serve it in lettuce wraps for a crunchy and kidney-friendly option.

4. **Hummus and Veggie Sandwich:** Spread low-sodium hummus on whole-grain bread and layer with sliced cucumber, tomatoes, and lettuce.

5. **Smoked Salmon and Cream Cheese Bagel:** Enjoy a classic combination of smoked salmon and low-sodium cream cheese on a whole-grain bagel. Add capers and red onion for extra flavor.

6. **Roast Beef and Horseradish Wrap:** Wrap thinly sliced roast beef with low-sodium horseradish, lettuce, and tomato in a whole-grain tortilla.

7. **Tuna Salad Lettuce Cups:** Make a kidney-friendly tuna salad with low-sodium tuna, Greek yogurt, and diced vegetables. Serve in lettuce cups.

8. **Mediterranean Veggie Pita:** Stuff a whole-grain pita with kidney-friendly vegetables like cucumbers, cherry tomatoes, olives, and feta cheese.

9. **Grilled Portobello Mushroom Burger:** Grill portobello mushrooms and serve them as a burger with low-sodium condiments, lettuce, and tomato on a whole-grain bun.

10. **Caprese Sandwich:** Layer sliced tomatoes, fresh mozzarella, and basil on whole-grain bread. Drizzle with balsamic glaze for a kidney-friendly Caprese sandwich.

11. **Chicken Salad on Rye:** Prepare a low-sodium chicken salad with diced chicken, celery, and Greek yogurt. Spread it on whole-grain rye bread.

12. **Peanut Butter and Banana Wrap:** Spread low-sodium peanut butter on a whole-grain wrap, add sliced banana, and roll it up for a quick and tasty option.

13. **Veggie and Hummus Baguette:** Load a whole-grain baguette with kidney-friendly veggies and hummus for a satisfying and nutritious sandwich.

14. **Avocado and Tomato on Toast:** Mash avocado and spread it on whole-grain toast. Top with sliced tomatoes, salt-free seasoning, and a drizzle of olive oil.

15. **Turkey Cranberry Lettuce Wrap:** Wrap sliced turkey with cranberry sauce and lettuce in a whole-grain tortilla for a flavorful and low-sodium option.

Remember to adapt these sandwich options based on individual dietary needs and consult with healthcare professionals or registered dietitians for personalized guidance on renal-friendly meal options.

CHAPTER NINE
DELICIOUS DINNER

Grilled Protein with Flavorful Marinades

1. **Lemon Herb Chicken:** Marinade chicken breasts in a mixture of fresh lemon juice, minced garlic, rosemary, thyme, and olive oil before grilling.

2. **Balsamic Dijon Salmon:** Combine balsamic vinegar, Dijon mustard, minced garlic, and a touch of honey for a tangy marinade for grilled salmon.

3. **Teriyaki Tofu Skewers:** Marinate tofu cubes in a kidney-friendly teriyaki sauce made with low-sodium soy sauce, ginger, garlic, and a hint of brown sugar.

4. **Minty Yogurt Lamb Chops:** Mix plain Greek yogurt with mint, garlic, cumin, and coriander for a flavorful marinade for grilled lamb chops.

5. **Cilantro Lime Shrimp:** Combine fresh cilantro, lime juice, minced garlic, and olive oil for a zesty marinade for grilled shrimp.

6. **Rosemary Dijon Pork Tenderloin:** Create a marinade using Dijon mustard, chopped rosemary, garlic, and olive oil for grilled pork tenderloin.

7. **Ginger Sesame Chicken Skewers:** Marinate chicken skewers in a mixture of grated ginger, low-sodium soy sauce, sesame oil, and a touch of honey before grilling.

8. **Maple Mustard Turkey Burgers:** Mix together maple syrup, Dijon mustard, minced garlic, and thyme for a sweet and savory marinade for turkey burgers.

9. **Garlic Herb Swordfish:** Marinate swordfish steaks in a blend of minced garlic, fresh herbs (such as parsley and chives), lemon juice, and olive oil.

10. **Citrus Chipotle Shrimp:** Combine orange juice, chipotle peppers in adobo sauce, garlic, and olive oil for a spicy and citrusy marinade for grilled shrimp.

11. **Soy Ginger Beef Skewers:** Marinate beef skewers in a mixture of low-sodium soy sauce, grated ginger, garlic, and a touch of brown sugar for an Asian-inspired flavor.

12. **Lime Cumin Grilled Chicken Thighs:** Mix lime juice, ground cumin, minced garlic, and olive oil for a zesty marinade for grilled chicken thighs.

13. **Honey Mustard Glazed Salmon:** Create a sweet and tangy marinade for salmon using a blend of honey, Dijon mustard, minced garlic, and lemon juice.

14. **Lemon Rosemary Portobello Mushrooms:** Marinate portobello mushrooms in a mixture of fresh lemon juice, chopped rosemary, garlic, and olive oil before grilling.

15. **Miso Glazed Eggplant Steaks:** Make a marinade using white miso paste, rice vinegar, sesame oil, and a touch of maple syrup for grilled eggplant steaks.

Adjust these marinades based on individual dietary needs, and consult with healthcare professionals or registered dietitians for personalized guidance on renal-friendly meal options.

Pasta and Rice Dishes for Kidney

Pasta:

1. **Lemon Garlic Shrimp Pasta:** Toss whole-grain pasta with sautéed shrimp, minced garlic, fresh lemon juice, and kidney-friendly herbs.

2. **Tomato Basil Penne:** Cook whole-grain penne and toss it with a kidney-friendly tomato and basil sauce. Add grated Parmesan cheese in moderation.

3. **Mushroom Spinach Alfredo:** Make a kidney-friendly Alfredo sauce using low-fat cream, mushrooms, and spinach. Mix it with whole-grain fettuccine.

4. **Pesto Zucchini Noodles:** Spiralize zucchini into noodles and toss them with a kidney-friendly pesto made with basil, garlic, pine nuts, and olive oil.

5. **Eggplant and Tomato Rotini:** Roast eggplant and tomatoes, then mix them with

whole-grain rotini and a kidney-friendly marinara sauce.

6. **Chicken and Broccoli Rigatoni:** Combine whole-grain rigatoni with grilled chicken, steamed broccoli, and a kidney-friendly garlic sauce.

7. **Primavera Spaghetti Squash:** Roast spaghetti squash and mix it with kidney-friendly vegetables, olive oil, and herbs for a low-carb pasta alternative.

8. **Lentil Bolognese:** Make a kidney-friendly lentil Bolognese sauce and serve it over whole-grain spaghetti.

9. **Spinach and Tomato Orzo Salad:** Toss cooked orzo with fresh spinach, cherry tomatoes, olive oil, and kidney-friendly herbs for a refreshing salad.

10. **Shrimp Scampi Linguine:** Sauté shrimp in garlic, lemon juice, and white wine. Mix with

whole-grain linguine for a quick and flavorful dish.

Rice:

1. **Vegetable Fried Rice:** Stir-fry brown rice with kidney-friendly vegetables, tofu, and a low-sodium soy sauce for a nutritious fried rice.

2. **Mushroom Risotto:** Prepare a kidney-friendly mushroom risotto using arborio rice, low-sodium vegetable broth, and a touch of white wine.

3. **Lemon Herb Quinoa:** Cook quinoa and toss it with fresh lemon juice, kidney-friendly herbs, and sautéed vegetables.

4. **Greek Chickpea and Brown Rice Bowl:** Mix brown rice with chickpeas, cherry tomatoes, cucumber, feta cheese, and a kidney-friendly Greek dressing.

5. **Tomato Basil Rice Pilaf:** Sauté brown rice with diced tomatoes, basil, and low-sodium vegetable broth for a flavorful rice pilaf.

6. **Black Bean and Corn Quinoa Salad:** Combine cooked quinoa with black beans, corn, red onion, and a kidney-friendly lime dressing for a refreshing salad.

7. **Chicken and Vegetable Wild Rice:** Cook wild rice with grilled chicken, kidney-friendly vegetables, and a touch of olive oil.

8. **Butternut Squash Risotto:** Make a kidney-friendly risotto using butternut squash, arborio rice, and low-sodium vegetable broth.

9. **Lemon Garlic Shrimp and Brown Rice:** Sauté shrimp with garlic and lemon juice and serve over cooked brown rice for a quick and tasty meal.

10. **Mediterranean Quinoa Bowl:** Create a bowl with cooked quinoa, kidney-friendly vegetables, olives, feta cheese, and a lemon-tahini dressing.

Adapt these recipes based on individual dietary needs and consult with healthcare professionals or registered dietitians for personalized guidance on renal-friendly meal options.

Salads with Kidney-Friendly Ingredients

1. **Mixed Greens with Berries:** Combine mixed greens with kidney-friendly berries like strawberries, blueberries, and raspberries. Top with a light vinaigrette.

2. **Cucumber and Avocado Salad:** Toss sliced cucumbers and avocados with cherry tomatoes, red onion, and kidney-friendly herbs. Dress with olive oil and lemon juice.

3. **Greek Salad with Chickpeas:** Make a Greek salad with kidney-friendly ingredients like cherry tomatoes, cucumber, feta cheese, olives,

and chickpeas. Dress with a light Greek vinaigrette.

4. **Quinoa and Vegetable Salad:** Combine cooked quinoa with kidney-friendly vegetables like bell peppers, cherry tomatoes, and cucumbers. Drizzle with a lemon-tahini dressing.

5. **Caprese Salad with Basil:** Arrange sliced tomatoes, fresh mozzarella, and basil leaves on a plate. Drizzle with balsamic glaze for a kidney-friendly Caprese salad.

6. **Spinach and Strawberry Salad:** Mix fresh spinach with sliced strawberries, almonds (in moderation), and feta cheese. Dress with a kidney-friendly balsamic vinaigrette.

7. **Mango Black Bean Salad:** Toss black beans with diced mango, red onion, and cilantro. For added taste, pour in some lime juice.

8. **Broccoli and Walnut Salad:** Combine broccoli florets with kidney-friendly ingredients like walnuts, raisins, and a light yogurt dressing.

9. **Tuna and White Bean Salad:** Mix canned tuna with white beans, cherry tomatoes, red

onion, and parsley. Dress with olive oil and lemon juice.

10. **Asian Sesame Cabbage Salad:** Shred cabbage and carrots, then toss with kidney-friendly ingredients like edamame, sesame seeds, and a light soy-ginger dressing.

11. **Arugula and Watermelon Salad:** Combine arugula with chunks of watermelon, feta cheese (in moderation), and mint. Drizzle with a balsamic reduction.

12. **Chicken Caesar Salad:** Make a kidney-friendly Caesar salad with grilled chicken, romaine lettuce, cherry tomatoes, and a light Caesar dressing.

13. **Lentil and Tomato Salad:** Mix cooked lentils with diced tomatoes, cucumber, red onion, and kidney-friendly herbs. Dress with olive oil and red wine vinegar.

14. **Orange and Beet Salad:** Combine sliced beets with orange segments, arugula, and crumbled goat cheese (in moderation). Drizzle with a citrus vinaigrette.

15. **Walnut and Apple Spinach Salad:** Toss fresh spinach with sliced apples, walnuts, and kidney-friendly goat cheese. Dress with a light apple cider vinaigrette.

Remember to customize these salads based on individual dietary needs and consult with healthcare professionals or registered dietitians for personalized guidance on renal-friendly meal options.

CHAPTER TEN
SIDE DISHES AND SNACKS

Renal-Friendly Snacking

1. **Fresh Fruit Cups:** Enjoy kidney-friendly fruits like apple slices, grapes, or melon in portion-controlled cups.

2. **Vegetable Sticks with Hummus:** Dip kidney-friendly vegetables such as cucumber, bell pepper, and carrot sticks in a low-sodium hummus.

3. **Greek Yogurt Parfait:** Layer low-potassium Greek yogurt with kidney-friendly berries and a sprinkle of nuts (in moderation).

4. **Rice Cake with Almond Butter:** Spread almond butter on a rice cake for a satisfying and kidney-friendly snack.

5. **Cottage Cheese with Pineapple:** Pair low-phosphorus cottage cheese with diced pineapple for a tasty and protein-packed snack.

6. **Hard-Boiled Eggs:** Enjoy hard-boiled eggs as a protein-rich and kidney-friendly snack.

7. **Roasted Chickpeas:** Roast chickpeas with kidney-friendly spices like cumin and paprika for a crunchy and nutritious snack.

8. **Cheese and Whole-Grain Crackers:** Pair low-potassium cheese with whole-grain crackers for a satisfying and balanced snack.

9. **Popcorn with Herbs:** Air-pop popcorn and season it with kidney-friendly herbs like rosemary or thyme for a flavorful snack.

10. **Fresh Berries with Whipped Cream:** Top kidney-friendly berries with a dollop of low-potassium whipped cream for a sweet treat.

11. **Nuts Mix (in Moderation):** Create a mix of kidney-friendly nuts like almonds and walnuts with a touch of dried fruit.

12. **Yogurt and Berry Smoothie:** Blend low-potassium yogurt with kidney-friendly berries for a refreshing smoothie.

13. **Apple Slices with Nut Butter:** Slice apples and pair them with kidney-friendly nut butter for a satisfying and nutritious snack.

14. **Cherry Tomatoes with Mozzarella:** Enjoy cherry tomatoes with small portions of low-potassium mozzarella for a simple and tasty snack.

15. **Oatmeal Cookies (Low in Phosphorus):** Bake homemade oatmeal cookies using kidney-friendly ingredients and limited phosphorus.

Remember to monitor portion sizes and choose snacks that align with individual dietary needs. Consulting with healthcare professionals or registered dietitians is essential for personalized guidance on renal-friendly snacking.

Nuts and Seed Options

1. **Almonds:** Almonds are a good source of healthy fats and protein. Choose unsalted almonds for a kidney-friendly option.

2. **Walnuts:** Walnuts provide omega-3 fatty acids and can be a nutritious addition to your diet. Consume them in moderation.

3. **Pumpkin Seeds (Pepitas):** Pumpkin seeds are rich in iron and a kidney-friendly alternative. Roast them for a crunchy snack.

4. **Sunflower Seeds:** Sunflower seeds are a good source of vitamin E and healthy fats. Opt for unsalted sunflower seeds.

5. **Chia Seeds:** Chia seeds are high in fiber and can be added to smoothies, yogurt, or puddings for a kidney-friendly boost.

6. **Flaxseeds:** Ground flaxseeds are rich in omega-3 fatty acids and can be sprinkled on cereals or added to smoothies.

7. **Cashews:** Cashews are lower in phosphorus compared to some other nuts. Choose unsalted cashews for snacking.

8. **Brazil Nuts:** Selenium may be found in abundance in brazil nuts. Eat them in moderation as they contain selenium.

9. **Pistachios:** Pistachios are relatively lower in phosphorus compared to some other nuts. Choose unsalted pistachios.

10. **Hazelnuts:** Hazelnuts are a tasty and kidney-friendly option. Opt for unsalted hazelnuts for a snack.

11. **Pine Nuts:** Pine nuts are a good source of magnesium. Use them in moderation as a topping for salads or dishes.

12. **Sesame Seeds:** Sesame seeds are rich in nutrients and can be sprinkled on salads or used in cooking.

13. **Poppy Seeds:** Poppy seeds are a kidney-friendly option and can be added to baked goods or salads.

14. **Hemp Seeds:** Hemp seeds are rich in omega-3 fatty acids and protein. Blend them into shakes or scatter them over greens.

15. **Macadamia Nuts:** Macadamia nuts are lower in phosphorus compared to some other nuts. Enjoy them in moderation.

Always be mindful of portion sizes and consider your individual dietary restrictions. Consult with healthcare professionals or a registered dietitian for personalized guidance on incorporating nuts and seeds into a renal-friendly diet.

Healthy Sides for Kidney Health

1. **Steamed Asparagus:** Asparagus is a low-potassium vegetable that can be steamed and drizzled with a touch of olive oil.

2. **Roasted Brussels Sprouts:** Roast Brussels sprouts with kidney-friendly herbs and spices for a flavorful side dish.

3. **Cucumber and Tomato Salad:** Toss sliced cucumbers and tomatoes with kidney-friendly herbs, olive oil, and balsamic vinegar.

4. **Quinoa Pilaf:** Cook quinoa with low-potassium vegetables like bell peppers and peas for a nutritious side.

5. **Sautéed Spinach with Garlic:** Sauté spinach with minced garlic and a squeeze of lemon for a quick and healthy side.

6. **Baked Sweet Potato Wedges:** Bake sweet potato wedges with kidney-friendly spices like cinnamon and paprika.

7. **Green Bean Almondine:** Sauté green beans with slivered almonds and a splash of lemon juice for a crunchy side.

8. **Mashed Cauliflower:** Make a kidney-friendly alternative to mashed potatoes by mashing cauliflower with a touch of low-potassium milk.

9. **Brown Rice with Vegetables:** Mix cooked brown rice with kidney-friendly vegetables like carrots, peas, and corn for a wholesome side.

10. **Grilled Zucchini:** Grill zucchini slices and season them with kidney-friendly herbs and a drizzle of olive oil.

11. **Mushroom and Pea Risotto:** Prepare a kidney-friendly risotto with mushrooms, peas, and arborio rice using low-sodium vegetable broth.

12. **Baked Acorn Squash:** Roast acorn squash halves and drizzle with a touch of maple syrup for a sweet and savory side.

13. **Sautéed Kale with Lemon:** Sauté kale with garlic and finish with a squeeze of lemon juice for a nutritious side dish.

14. **Herbed Couscous:** Cook whole-grain couscous and toss it with kidney-friendly herbs, diced tomatoes, and cucumber.

15. **Roasted Eggplant:** Roast eggplant slices with kidney-friendly spices for a flavorful and low-calorie side.

Remember to tailor these side dishes to individual dietary needs and consult with healthcare professionals or a registered dietitian for personalized guidance on incorporating healthy sides into a renal-friendly diet.

Renal-Friendly Salsa and Guacamole

Ingredients:

- 1 cup diced tomatoes (choose lower potassium varieties)
- 1/2 cup diced cucumber
- 1/4 cup finely chopped red onion
- 1/4 cup chopped fresh cilantro
- 1 clove garlic, minced
- 1 tablespoon lime juice
- Salt and pepper to taste

Instructions:

1. In a bowl, combine diced tomatoes, cucumber, red onion, cilantro, and minced garlic.

2. Add lime juice and gently toss the ingredients.

3. Season with salt and pepper to taste.

4. Before serving, let the food cool for at least half an hour in the refrigerator.

5. Serve with kidney-friendly tortilla chips or as a topping for grilled chicken or fish.

Renal-Friendly Guacamole Recipe:
Ingredients:
- 2 ripe avocados, peeled and mashed
- 1/4 cup diced red onion
- 1 small tomato, diced (choose lower potassium varieties)
- 1 clove garlic, minced
- 1 tablespoon lime juice
- 1 tablespoon chopped fresh cilantro
- Salt and pepper to taste

Instructions:
1. Mash the ripe avocados in a bowl.
2. Add diced red onion, diced tomato, minced garlic, lime juice, and chopped cilantro to the mashed avocados.
3. Mix until well combined.
4. To taste, add salt and pepper for seasoning.
5. Chill in the refrigerator for at least 30 minutes to let the flavors meld.
6. Serve with kidney-friendly tortilla chips or as a topping for tacos or grilled proteins.

These recipes are tailored to be kidney-friendly, but it's crucial to consider individual dietary needs and consult with healthcare professionals or a registered dietitian for personalized guidance on renal-friendly meal options.

CHAPTER ELEVEN
DESSERTS FOR RENAL DIETS
Low-Phosphorus Sweet Treats

1. **Frozen Banana Bites:** Dip banana slices in melted dark chocolate (low in phosphorus) and freeze for a tasty and kidney-friendly dessert.

2. **Baked Apples:** Core apples and fill the center with a mixture of cinnamon and a touch of honey. Bake until tender for a warm and sweet treat.

3. **Berry Sorbet:** Blend kidney-friendly berries with a splash of water and a touch of honey. Freeze the mixture for a refreshing sorbet.

4. **Chia Seed Pudding:** Mix chia seeds with low-potassium milk and sweeten with a small amount of honey. Let it sit until it thickens for a pudding-like treat.

5. **Peach Slices with Almond Butter:** Enjoy sliced peaches with a smear of almond butter for a satisfying and low-phosphorus dessert.

6. **Coconut Milk Rice Pudding:** Make rice pudding using coconut milk and sweeten with a small amount of sugar or honey for a creamy and flavorful dessert.

7. **Watermelon Cubes:** Fresh watermelon cubes are a hydrating and low-phosphorus sweet option.

8. **Gingered Mango:** Toss mango cubes with a sprinkle of ginger for a sweet and slightly spicy flavor.

9. **Angel Food Cake with Berries:** Top a slice of angel food cake with kidney-friendly berries for a light and delicious dessert.

10. **Lemon Sorbet:** Make a simple lemon sorbet using lemon juice, water, and a touch of sweetener. Freeze until solid.

11. **Cinnamon Baked Pears:** Slice pears and sprinkle with cinnamon before baking until tender for a warm and comforting treat.

12. **Vanilla Pudding with Fresh Strawberries:** Choose a low-phosphorus vanilla pudding and top it with fresh strawberries for a classic and kidney-friendly dessert.

13. **Homemade Fruit Salad:** Combine kidney-friendly fruits like melons, grapes, and berries for a refreshing and low-phosphorus fruit salad.

14. **Pistachio-Free Ice Cream:** Opt for pistachio-free ice cream alternatives that use low-phosphorus ingredients for a cool treat.

15. **Date and Nut Bites:** Blend dates and kidney-friendly nuts into bite-sized energy balls for a sweet and nutritious snack.

Always consider individual dietary needs and consult with healthcare professionals or a registered dietitian for personalized guidance on incorporating low-phosphorus sweet treats into a renal-friendly diet.

Fruit-Based Desserts

1. **Baked Cinnamon Apples:** Core and slice apples, sprinkle with cinnamon, and bake until tender for a warm and comforting treat.

2. **Mixed Berry Parfait:** Layer kidney-friendly berries with low-phosphorus yogurt or whipped cream for a delightful parfait.

3. **Grilled Pineapple with Honey:** Grill pineapple slices and drizzle with a touch of honey for a sweet and caramelized dessert.

4. **Citrus Salad with Mint:** Combine citrus segments (like oranges and grapefruits) and mint leaves for a refreshing and vitamin C-rich dessert.

5. **Fruit Kabobs:** Skewer kidney-friendly fruits like melons, grapes, and berries for a fun and colorful dessert.

6. **Mango Sorbet:** Blend ripe mango with a splash of water and freeze for a tropical and kidney-friendly sorbet.

7. **Poached Pears:** Poach pears in a mixture of water, cinnamon, and a touch of sweetener for an elegant and tender dessert.

8. **Papaya Boat:** Scoop out the seeds of a papaya and fill the center with a mixture of diced fruits for a unique and tropical dessert.

9. **Fruit Salsa with Cinnamon Chips:** Dice kidney-friendly fruits and mix them with a squeeze of lime juice. Serve with homemade cinnamon chips.

10. **Peach Melba:** Top sliced peaches with kidney-friendly raspberry sauce and a dollop of low-phosphorus whipped cream.

11. **Banana "Ice Cream":** Freeze banana slices and blend until creamy for a simple and naturally sweet ice cream alternative.

12. **Strawberry Shortcake:** Layer sliced strawberries over a kidney-friendly shortcake or angel food cake, and top with low-phosphorus whipped cream.

13. **Blueberry Lemon Yogurt Popsicles:** Mix blueberries and lemon-flavored low-phosphorus yogurt, then freeze in popsicle molds for a refreshing dessert.

14. **Cherry Almond Compote:** Cook cherries with a touch of almond extract for a flavorful compote. Serve over low-phosphorus vanilla ice cream.

15. **Melon Balls with Mint:** Use a melon baller to create colorful balls of kidney-friendly melons. Garnish with fresh mint for a light and refreshing dessert.

Always consider individual dietary needs and consult with healthcare professionals or a registered dietitian for personalized guidance on incorporating fruit-based desserts into a renal-friendly diet.

CHAPTER TWELVE
BEVERAGES FOR KIDNEY HEALTH
Hydration Tips

1. **Monitor Fluid Intake:** Keep track of your fluid intake to ensure you're meeting your hydration needs without overloading your kidneys.

2. **Sip Throughout the Day:** Drink fluids gradually throughout the day rather than consuming large amounts at once. This helps your body absorb fluids more efficiently.

3. **Choose Kidney-Friendly Beverages:** Opt for kidney-friendly beverages such as water, herbal teas, and clear broths. Limit or avoid drinks high in phosphorus, potassium, and sodium.

4. **Limit Caffeine and Sugar:** Reduce intake of caffeinated and sugary beverages, as excessive consumption may contribute to dehydration.

5. **Add Flavor to Water:** Infuse water with natural flavors by adding slices of citrus fruits, cucumber, mint, or berries for a refreshing taste.

6. **Be Mindful of Alcohol:** Consume alcohol in moderation, as excessive alcohol intake can contribute to dehydration.

7. **Eat Hydrating Foods:** Include water-rich foods in your diet, such as watermelon, cucumber, celery, and oranges, to contribute to overall hydration.

8. **Use a Straw:** Drinking through a straw can make it easier to manage fluid intake and may be helpful for those with difficulty swallowing.

9. **Manage Salt Intake:** Control your salt intake to help maintain fluid balance. High sodium levels can contribute to dehydration.

10. **Stay Cool in Hot Weather:** Increase fluid intake during hot weather or if you're engaging in physical activities that cause you to sweat.

11. **Consider Individual Needs:** Tailor your fluid intake to your individual needs, considering factors such as age, weight, activity level, and overall health.

12. **Consult with Healthcare Professionals:** Seek guidance from healthcare professionals or a registered dietitian to determine personalized hydration goals based on your specific health conditions.

13. **Monitor Urine Color:** Pay attention to the color of your urine. In general, pale yellow or light straw color indicates that you are adequately hydrated.

14. **Space Out Medications:** If you're on medications that affect fluid balance, work with your healthcare provider to schedule them in a way that supports proper hydration.

15. **Listen to Your Body:** Be aware of the cues that your body sends forth. Thirst is a natural indicator that it's time to drink water, so respond to those cues.

Remember, individual hydration needs may vary, and it's crucial to consult with healthcare professionals or a registered dietitian for personalized guidance on maintaining proper hydration, especially if you have kidney-related concerns.

Drinks to Avoid and Embrace

1. **Soda and Carbonated Drinks:** High in phosphorus and often contain added sugars, which can be detrimental to kidney health.

2. **Energy Drinks:** Typically high in caffeine and may contain excessive sugars and additives.

3. **Sports Drinks:** Often contain added sugars and electrolytes that can be unnecessary unless engaged in vigorous physical activity.

4. **Aloe Vera Juice:** Some aloe vera juice products can contain compounds that may be harmful to the kidneys, so it's advisable to consult with a healthcare professional.

5. **High-Potassium Fruit Juices:** Juices from fruits high in potassium, such as oranges and bananas, may need to be limited for individuals with kidney issues.

6. **Vegetable Juice Blends:** Certain vegetable juice blends may have high potassium content, so it's essential to be mindful of the ingredients.

7. **Alcohol:** Excessive alcohol consumption can contribute to dehydration and stress the kidneys. Moderation is key.

8. **Sweetened Iced Tea:** Pre-packaged or commercially sweetened iced teas can contain high levels of added sugars.

9. **Flavored Waters with Additives:** Flavored waters may contain artificial additives and sugars that can be detrimental to kidney health.

Kidney-Friendly Drinks to Embrace:

1. **Water:** The best choice for staying hydrated without adding extra nutrients that could strain the kidneys.

2. **Herbal Teas:** Unsweetened herbal teas, such as chamomile or peppermint, can be soothing and hydrating.

3. **Freshly Squeezed Juice in Moderation:** Freshly squeezed juices from lower-potassium fruits like apples or berries can be enjoyed in moderation.

4. **Cranberry Juice:** Unsweetened cranberry juice may be beneficial for urinary tract health but should be consumed in moderation.

5. **Coconut Water:** A natural source of electrolytes, coconut water can be a hydrating option.

6. **Lemonade (Made with Real Lemons):** Homemade lemonade with real lemons and a touch of sweetener can be kidney-friendly.

7. **Diluted Fruit Juices:** Diluting fruit juices with water can reduce their potassium and sugar content.

8. **Clear Broth:** Clear broths like chicken or vegetable broth can contribute to hydration.

9. **Almond Milk (Low-Potassium Varieties):** Almond milk in low-potassium varieties can be a suitable dairy alternative.

10. **Iced Herbal Tea:** Unsweetened iced herbal teas, like hibiscus or green tea, can be a refreshing choice.

Remember, individual dietary needs can vary, and it's essential to consult with healthcare professionals or a registered dietitian for personalized guidance on beverages that align with your kidney health.

Smoothies and Drinks with Limited Phosphorus

1. **Berry Blast Smoothie:** Blend a mix of kidney-friendly berries (like blueberries and strawberries) with almond milk and ice.

2. **Pineapple Mint Cooler:** Blend pineapple chunks, fresh mint leaves, and coconut water for a tropical and refreshing smoothie.

3. **Green Goddess Smoothie:** Combine spinach, cucumber, celery, and a splash of low-potassium fruit juice for a nutrient-packed green smoothie.

4. **Peachy Keen Smoothie:** Blend peaches, low-potassium yogurt, and a hint of vanilla for a smooth and peach-flavored treat.

5. **Cucumber Melon Refresher:** Blend cucumber, honeydew melon, and mint with ice for a hydrating and low-phosphorus drink.

6. **Avocado Berry Delight:** Mix avocado, low-potassium berries, and almond milk for a creamy and nutrient-rich smoothie.

7. **Carrot Ginger Zinger:** Blend carrots, ginger, and orange segments with ice for a zesty and low-phosphorus smoothie.

8. **Watermelon Lime Splash:** Combine watermelon chunks, lime juice, and a splash of water for a light and hydrating smoothie.

9. **Coconut Berry Bliss:** Blend mixed berries with coconut water and a scoop of low-phosphorus protein powder for a tropical twist.

10. **Cherry Almond Dream:** Mix cherries, almond milk, and a small amount of almond butter for a flavorful and low-phosphorus smoothie.

Low-Phosphorus Drinks:

1. **Iced Hibiscus Tea:** Brew hibiscus tea, chill, and serve over ice for a refreshing and low-phosphorus drink.

2. **Ginger Lemonade:** Make lemonade with fresh lemon juice, water, and a touch of grated ginger for a zesty beverage.

3. **Cranberry Spritzer:** Dilute unsweetened cranberry juice with sparkling water for a tart and bubbly low-phosphorus drink.

4. **Minty Iced Green Tea:** Brew green tea, add fresh mint leaves, and chill for a cool and antioxidant-rich beverage.

5. **Sparkling Water with Citrus Slices:** Enjoy plain sparkling water with slices of lemon, lime, or orange for a simple and hydrating option.

6. **Herbal Infused Water:** Create your own infused water with herbs like mint, basil, or rosemary along with slices of cucumber or berries.

7. **Apple Cider Cooler:** Dilute low-potassium apple cider with water and add ice for a fall-inspired and low-phosphorus drink.

8. **Blueberry Lemon Sparkler:** Mix blueberry juice (low-potassium) with sparkling water and a squeeze of lemon for a flavorful and fizzy option.

9. **Peach Iced Tea:** Brew low-phosphorus peach tea and chill for a sweet and peachy iced tea.

10. **Cherry Limeade:** Combine fresh lime juice, water, and a small amount of unsweetened cherry juice for a tangy and low-phosphorus drink.

Remember to tailor these recipes to individual dietary needs and consult with healthcare professionals or a registered dietitian for personalized guidance on incorporating low-phosphorus smoothies and drinks into a renal-friendly diet.

Herbal Tea and Coffee Options

1. **Peppermint Tea:** Refreshing and caffeine-free, peppermint tea is a soothing option for any time of day.

2. **Chamomile Tea:** Known for its calming properties, chamomile tea is a gentle and relaxing choice.

3. **Hibiscus Tea:** Hibiscus tea is tart and fruity, making it a flavorful and low-phosphorus option.

4. **Ginger Tea:** Brewed from fresh ginger, this tea has a warming and spicy flavor with potential anti-inflammatory benefits.

5. **Lemon Balm Tea:** Lemon balm tea has a mild citrus flavor and is often used for relaxation and stress relief.

6. **Rooibos Tea:** Naturally caffeine-free, rooibos tea has a sweet and nutty flavor, making it a great alternative to traditional tea.

7. **Nettle Tea:** Despite its name, nettle tea is not high in oxalates and can be a nutritious and earthy option.

8. **Dandelion Root Tea:** Dandelion root tea has a slightly bitter taste and is believed to support kidney health.

9. **Lavender Tea:** Lavender tea offers a floral and aromatic experience, known for its potential calming effects.

10. **Rosehip Tea:** Rich in vitamin C, rosehip tea has a fruity and tangy flavor.

Low-Phosphorus Coffee Options:

1. **Cold Brew Coffee:** Cold brew coffee tends to be lower in acidity and can be a smoother option for those with sensitive stomachs.

2. **Decaffeinated Coffee:** Opt for decaffeinated coffee to reduce caffeine intake, especially if advised by healthcare professionals.

3. **Instant Coffee:** Choose instant coffee without added phosphorus-containing additives for a quick and convenient option.

4. **Black Coffee:** Plain black coffee is naturally low in phosphorus and can be enjoyed in moderation.

5. **Coffee Alternatives:** Explore coffee alternatives like chicory root coffee or herbal coffee blends for a caffeine-free option.

6. **Almond Milk Latte:** Create a low-phosphorus latte using almond milk and decaffeinated coffee.

7. **Coconut Milk Coffee:** Use coconut milk as a dairy alternative for a creamy and low-phosphorus coffee option.

8. **Herbal Infused Coffee:** Experiment with herbal infusions like cinnamon or cardamom in your coffee for added flavor without extra phosphorus.

9. **Vanilla Almond Iced Coffee:** Make a refreshing iced coffee using decaffeinated coffee, almond milk, and a touch of vanilla.

10. **Mocha Smoothie:** Blend decaffeinated coffee with low-phosphorus chocolate protein powder, ice, and a non-dairy milk for a flavorful mocha smoothie.

Remember to monitor your overall phosphorus intake, as additives or flavorings in commercial teas and coffees can contribute to phosphorus levels. Always consult with healthcare professionals or a registered dietitian for personalized guidance on incorporating herbal teas and coffee into a renal-friendly diet.

CHAPTER THIRTEEN
SAMPLE MEAL PLANS

4 Weeks Meal Plans

Renal-Friendly 4-Week Meal Plan:

Week 1:

Day 1:

- **Breakfast:** Oatmeal with sliced strawberries and a drizzle of honey.
- **Lunch:** Turkey and vegetable wrap with a side of mixed greens.
- **Dinner:** quinoa, Brussels sprouts, and baked chicken breast.

Day 2:

- **Breakfast:** Greek yogurt parfait with low-potassium berries and a sprinkle of granola.
- **Lunch:** Lentil soup with a whole-grain roll.
- **Dinner:** Grilled salmon with sweet potato wedges and sautéed spinach.

Day 3:

- **Breakfast:** Scrambled eggs with sautéed mushrooms and whole-grain toast.
- **Lunch:** Quinoa salad with kidney-friendly vegetables.
- **Dinner:** steamed broccoli and brown rice with stir-fried tofu.

Day 4:

- **Breakfast:** Smoothie with banana, blueberries, almond milk, and low-phosphorus protein powder.
- **Lunch:** Caprese salad with low-potassium mozzarella, tomatoes, and basil.
- **Dinner:** Baked cod with quinoa pilaf and green beans.

Day 5:

- **Breakfast:** Cottage cheese with sliced peaches and a sprinkle of chopped almonds.
- **Lunch:** Chickpea salad with mixed greens, olives, and feta cheese (in moderation).

- **Dinner:** Stir-fried vegetables and beef over brown rice.

Day 6:
- **Breakfast:** Avocado and cherry tomatoes on whole grain bread.
- **Lunch:** Spinach and feta omelet with a side of whole-grain crackers.
- **Dinner:** Grilled chicken skewers with vegetable kebabs and couscous.

Day 7:
- **Breakfast:** Smoothie bowl with blended berries, banana, and low-phosphorus granola.
- **Lunch:** Egg salad sandwich on whole-grain bread with a side of carrot sticks.
- **Dinner:** Shrimp and vegetable kebabs with quinoa and a side of asparagus.

Weeks 2-4:

Repeat the weekly meal plan, making small variations in ingredients and preparation methods to add variety. Consider incorporating seasonal produce and experimenting with herbs and spices for flavor. Monitor portion sizes and consult with healthcare professionals or a registered dietitian for any necessary adjustments based on individual needs.

Remember to stay hydrated and make adjustments to the meal plan as needed to accommodate any specific dietary requirements or recommendations from healthcare professionals.

Adjusting for Dietary Preferences

Renal-Friendly 4-Week Meal Plan with Adjustments for Dietary Preferences:

Week 1:

Day 1:

- **Breakfast:** Almond milk, chia seeds, and mixed berries for overnight oats.
- **Lunch:** Chickpea and avocado wrap with a side of hummus and vegetable sticks.
- **Dinner:** Baked tofu with quinoa and roasted Brussels sprouts.

Day 2:

- **Breakfast:** Smoothie with banana, spinach, almond butter, and low-phosphorus protein powder.
- **Lunch:** Mediterranean quinoa salad with olives, tomatoes, and feta cheese (in moderation).
- **Dinner:** Grilled portobello mushrooms with sweet potato wedges and sautéed spinach.

Day 3:

- **Breakfast:** Avocado toast with cherry tomatoes and a sprinkle of hemp seeds on whole-grain bread.
- **Lunch:** Brown rice and vegetable curry with lentils.
- **Dinner:** Teriyaki tempeh with quinoa and steamed broccoli.

Day 4:

- **Breakfast:** Greek yogurt parfait with low-potassium fruits, granola, and a drizzle of maple syrup.
- **Lunch:** Caprese-style quinoa bowl with low-potassium mozzarella, tomatoes, and basil.
- **Dinner:** Baked cod with wild rice pilaf and green beans.

Day 5:
- **Breakfast:** Almond milk chia pudding with sliced peaches and a sprinkle of almonds.
- **Lunch:** Spinach and mushroom whole-grain wrap with a side of mixed greens.
- **Dinner:** Stir-fried seitan with brown rice and a variety of kidney-friendly vegetables.

Day 6:
- **Breakfast:** Vegan protein smoothie with almond milk, banana, berries, and a scoop of plant-based protein powder.
- **Lunch:** Quinoa and black bean stuffed bell peppers with a side of guacamole.
- **Dinner:** Grilled vegetable skewers with quinoa and a tangy balsamic glaze.

Day 7:

- **Breakfast:** Smoothie bowl with blended mango, pineapple, and coconut milk, topped with shredded coconut.
- **Lunch:** Vegan chickpea salad sandwich on whole-grain bread with a side of carrot sticks.
- **Dinner:** Lentil and vegetable kebabs with couscous and a lemon tahini dressing.

Weeks 2-4:

Adapt the weekly meal plan by continuing to explore plant-based protein sources, incorporating different grains and legumes, and varying the types of fruits and vegetables used. Adjust seasonings and herbs to suit taste preferences. Always consider individual dietary needs and consult with healthcare professionals or a registered dietitian for personalized guidance.

CHAPTER FOURTEEN
DINING OUT ON A RENAL DIET
Tips for Eating at Restaurants

1. **Plan Ahead:** Check the restaurant's menu online before going to choose options that align with a renal-friendly diet.

2. **Communicate Dietary Needs:** Inform your server about any dietary restrictions or preferences, such as a need for low-sodium or phosphorus options.

3. **Ask for Modifications:** Don't hesitate to ask for modifications to dishes, such as requesting sauces or dressings on the side or choosing grilled instead of fried options.

4. **Choose Simple Preparations:** Opt for simple cooking methods like grilling, steaming, or baking, which can be healthier and easier to adapt to a renal-friendly diet.

5. **Be Mindful of Portions:** Restaurant portions are often larger than necessary. Consider sharing a dish or asking for a take-out container to save part of your meal for later.

6. **Select Lean Proteins:** Choose lean protein sources like grilled chicken, fish, or tofu. Avoid heavily processed or cured meats.

7. **Limit High-Potassium Foods:** Be cautious with high-potassium foods like tomatoes, potatoes, and bananas. Ask for substitutions or adjustments if needed.

8. **Control Sodium Intake:** Ask for dishes with less salt or request that the chef go easy on salt during preparation.

9. **Opt for Fresh Sides:** Choose fresh, steamed, or sautéed vegetables as side dishes instead of those that are canned or heavily seasoned.

10. **Skip or Modify Appetizers:n**Appetizers can be high in sodium and phosphorus. Consider skipping them or choosing simpler options like a green salad.

11. **Watch for Hidden Sodium:** Be aware of hidden sources of sodium, such as sauces, dressings, and processed foods. Ask for these to be served on the side.

12. **Hydrate Wisely:** Choose water or other kidney-friendly beverages instead of sugary drinks or those high in caffeine.

13. **Ask for Nutrition Information:** Some restaurants provide nutritional information upon request, which can help you make more informed choices.

14. **Bring Medications if Needed:** If you have medications related to your kidney condition, make sure to bring them with you and take them as prescribed.

15. **Enjoy Dessert in Moderation:** If you're in the mood for dessert, consider sharing with others or choosing a small portion of a kidney-friendly option.

Remember to be proactive, ask questions, and prioritize your health when dining out. If uncertain about menu options, don't hesitate to consult with healthcare professionals or a registered dietitian for guidance.

Navigating Menus for Kidney Health

1. **Prioritize Protein:** Choose lean protein sources like grilled chicken, fish, or tofu. Avoid processed or cured meats, which may be high in sodium.

2. **Control Sodium Intake:** Be mindful of high-sodium options. Opt for dishes with less added salt, and ask if the chef can prepare your meal with minimal salt.

3. **Choose Grilled or Baked:** Opt for grilled or baked dishes instead of fried options. This reduces unnecessary fat and calorie intake.

4. **Be Cautious with Sauces and Dressings:** Request sauces and dressings on the side to control your intake. Many restaurant sauces can be high in sodium and phosphorus.

5. **Limit High-Potassium Foods:** Be aware of high-potassium foods like tomatoes, potatoes, and bananas. Consider choosing alternatives or asking for substitutions.

6. **Embrace Vegetables:** Include a variety of kidney-friendly vegetables in your meals. Choose fresh, steamed, or sautéed options over canned or heavily seasoned varieties.

7. **Watch Portion Sizes:** Restaurant portions are often larger than necessary. Consider sharing a dish, asking for a half portion, or saving part of your meal for later.

8. **Check for Nutrition Information:** Some restaurants provide nutritional information for their menu items. Use this information to make informed choices.

9. **Consider Customization:** Don't hesitate to customize your order based on your dietary needs. Most restaurants are willing to accommodate requests.

10. **Stay Hydrated:** Choose water or other kidney-friendly beverages. Limit sugary drinks and those high in caffeine.

11. **Look for Kidney-Friendly Sides:** Choose sides like steamed or roasted vegetables, rice, or small salads. Avoid sides that may be high in sodium or phosphorus.

12. **Explore Plant-Based Options:** Plant-based proteins can be kidney-friendly. Consider dishes with beans, lentils, or tofu as alternatives.

13. **Moderate Dessert Intake:** If you have a sweet tooth, consider sharing dessert or choosing small portions of kidney-friendly options.

14. **Ask for Recommendations:** If you're unsure about menu choices, don't hesitate to ask your server for recommendations or modifications based on your dietary needs.

15. **Be Mindful of Beverages:** Choose beverages with no or low added sugars. Water, herbal teas, and other kidney-friendly options are ideal.

Remember, everyone's dietary needs are unique. Consult with healthcare professionals or a registered dietitian for personalized guidance on navigating menus and making choices that support your kidney health.

CHAPTER FIFTEEN
MANAGING SPECIAL DIETARY CONSIDERATIONS

Diabetes and Kidney Health

1. **Control Blood Sugar Levels:** Maintain blood glucose levels within the target range to reduce the risk of kidney complications. Regular monitoring and adherence to a diabetes management plan are crucial.

2. **Monitor Blood Pressure:** Keep blood pressure under control. High blood pressure can strain the kidneys, so regularly check and manage blood pressure levels.

3. **Follow a Kidney-Friendly Diet:** Adopt a diet that is not only suitable for diabetes but also supports kidney health. This may include controlling phosphorus, potassium, and sodium intake.

4. **Limit Phosphorus Intake:.**Be mindful of phosphorus in the diet. Choose low-phosphorus foods and consider working with a dietitian to create a balanced meal plan.

5. **Control Potassium Intake:** Manage potassium intake, especially if kidney function is compromised. Choose low-potassium foods and monitor levels as advised by healthcare professionals.

6. **Manage Sodium Intake:** Control sodium intake to help regulate blood pressure. Choose fresh, whole foods and limit processed and packaged items.

7. **Stay Hydrated:** Maintain proper hydration. Drinking enough water is essential for kidney health and can also help manage blood sugar levels.

8. **Regular Exercise:** Engage in regular physical activity. Exercise can help control blood sugar, manage weight, and promote overall cardiovascular health.

9. **Medication Adherence:** Take diabetes medications as prescribed by healthcare professionals. Adherence is vital for maintaining stable blood sugar levels.

10. **Quit Smoking:** If applicable, quit smoking. Smoking can worsen kidney damage and increase the risk of cardiovascular complications associated with diabetes.

11. **Limit Alcohol Consumption:** Consume alcohol in moderation, as excessive alcohol intake can impact blood sugar levels and overall health.

12. **Regular Medical Checkups:** Attend regular checkups with healthcare professionals to monitor kidney function, blood sugar levels, and overall health.

13. **Weight Management:** Maintain a healthy weight through a balanced diet and regular exercise. Weight management is crucial for both diabetes and kidney health.

14. **Consider Medications with Nephroprotective Effects:** Some medications used to manage diabetes may have additional nephroprotective effects. Discuss these options with healthcare professionals.

15. **Educate Yourself:** Stay informed about diabetes and kidney health. Understanding the interplay between these conditions empowers you to make informed lifestyle choices.

Individuals with diabetes should work closely with their healthcare team, including a registered dietitian, to create a personalized plan that addresses both diabetes management and kidney health. Regular monitoring and proactive lifestyle choices are key components of comprehensive care.

Hypertension and the Renal Diet

1. **Reduce Sodium Intake:** Limiting sodium is crucial for managing hypertension. Choose fresh, whole foods over processed ones, and be mindful of added salt in cooking and at the table.

2. **Focus on Fresh Fruits and Vegetables:** Include a variety of fresh fruits and vegetables in your diet. These are rich in nutrients and antioxidants while being naturally low in sodium.

3. **Choose Lean Proteins:** Opt for lean protein sources like skinless poultry, fish, tofu, and legumes. Limit processed and high-fat meats, which can contribute to hypertension.

4. **Control Phosphorus and Potassium Intake:** Work with a dietitian to manage phosphorus and potassium levels. High levels of these minerals can impact blood pressure and kidney health.

5. **Moderate Protein Intake:** While protein is essential, excessive protein intake may affect blood pressure. Work with healthcare professionals to determine an appropriate protein level for your individual needs.

6. **Stay Hydrated:** Drink plenty of water. Staying well-hydrated helps maintain overall health and can support healthy blood pressure levels.

7. **Limit Caffeine Intake:** While moderate caffeine intake is generally safe, excessive amounts may contribute to hypertension. Be mindful of your caffeine consumption from coffee, tea, and other sources.

8. **Maintain a Healthy Weight:** Losing excess weight can significantly impact blood pressure. Adopting a renal-friendly diet, combined with regular physical activity, supports weight management.

9. **Increase Fiber Intake:** Fiber-rich foods, such as whole grains, fruits, and vegetables, can contribute to heart health and help regulate blood pressure.

10. **Manage Stress:** Practice stress management techniques like deep breathing, meditation, or yoga. Chronic stress can contribute to hypertension.

11. **Limit Alcohol Consumption:** If you choose to drink alcohol, do so in moderation. Excessive alcohol intake can raise blood pressure and impact kidney function.

12. **Avoid High-Potassium Foods:** If your renal diet requires potassium restriction, be cautious with high-potassium foods, as elevated potassium levels can contribute to hypertension.

13. **Regular Exercise:** Engage in regular physical activity. Exercise not only supports weight management but also helps regulate blood pressure.

14. **Medication Adherence:** Take prescribed blood pressure medications as directed by healthcare professionals. Adherence to medication is crucial for controlling hypertension.

15. **Regular Monitoring:** Regularly monitor your blood pressure at home and attend scheduled checkups with healthcare professionals. This ensures timely adjustments to your management plan.

It is noteworthy that nutritional requirements differ across individuals. Obtain advice from medical specialists or a qualified dietitian to develop a customised renal diet plan that takes kidney health and hypertension into account. Good management requires regular contact with your healthcare team.

CHAPTER SIXTEEN
FREQUENTLY ASKED QUESTIONS
Common Concerns about Renal Diets

1. **Limited Food Options:** Some individuals worry that a renal diet restricts too many food options. However, with guidance from a dietitian, it's possible to enjoy a diverse and satisfying range of foods within the prescribed restrictions.

2. **Nutrient Deficiency:** Concerns about nutrient deficiency may arise due to dietary restrictions. However, a well-planned renal diet, often with the guidance of a dietitian, can meet nutritional needs while managing kidney health.

3. **Taste and Flavor:** There's a perception that renal diets may be bland. With creative cooking techniques, herbs, and spices, flavorful meals can be prepared within the constraints of a renal-friendly diet.

4. **Social Challenges:** Participating in social events may pose challenges, as some traditional dishes may not align with renal dietary

guidelines. Open communication with hosts and careful menu planning can help address this concern.

5. **Meal Preparation Time:** Individuals may worry about the time and effort required to prepare renal-friendly meals. However, with proper planning and simple cooking techniques, it's possible to create nutritious meals efficiently.

6. **Impact on Quality of Life:** Some individuals fear that a renal diet may negatively impact their quality of life. However, adapting to dietary changes and focusing on delicious, kidney-friendly options can enhance overall well-being.

7. **Social Isolation:** Concerns about feeling isolated or different during meals with others may arise. Communicating dietary needs and finding common ground in food choices can help mitigate this concern.

8. **Dietary Monotony:** The perception that a renal diet involves repetitive meals can be a concern. A dietitian can assist in creating varied meal plans, ensuring a balance of nutrients while avoiding monotony.

9. **Difficulty Dining Out:** Individuals may worry about challenges when dining out. However, with proactive communication with restaurant staff and making informed menu choices, it's possible to enjoy restaurant meals within renal dietary guidelines.

10. **Impact on Mental Health:** Managing dietary restrictions can impact mental health. Seeking support from healthcare professionals, dietitians, and support groups can provide coping strategies and emotional support.

11. **Concerns About Protein Intake:** Some individuals worry about getting enough protein while following a renal diet. A dietitian can help plan a diet that meets protein needs without overloading the kidneys.

12. **Balancing Multiple Health Conditions:** Managing multiple health conditions alongside kidney issues can be challenging. Collaborative care involving various healthcare professionals helps create comprehensive and coordinated plans.

13. **Misinformation:** Concerns may arise from misinformation about renal diets. It's crucial to consult with trusted healthcare professionals or dietitians to receive accurate and personalized guidance.

Addressing concerns and misconceptions about renal diets requires open communication with healthcare professionals. A registered dietitian specializing in renal nutrition can play a key role in dispelling myths, providing accurate information, and helping individuals navigate their unique dietary needs.

Troubleshooting Tips

1. Concern: Limited Food Options

Tip: Collaborate with a registered dietitian to explore a variety of kidney-friendly foods and recipes. Get creative with herbs and spices to enhance flavors.

2. Concern: Nutrient Deficiency

Tip: Work closely with healthcare professionals and dietitians to ensure your renal diet meets all nutritional needs. Consider supplements if necessary, under professional guidance.

3. Concern: Taste and Flavor

Tip: Experiment with herbs, spices, and low-sodium seasonings to add flavor to meals. Try new cooking methods like grilling or roasting for added taste.

4. Concern: Social Challenges

Tip: Communicate your dietary needs with friends and family. Offer to bring a kidney-friendly dish to gatherings, ensuring you can enjoy meals together.

5. Concern: Meal Preparation Time

Tip: Plan your meals in advance and explore quick and easy renal-friendly recipes. Batch cooking and meal prepping can save time during busy periods.

6. **Concern: Impact on Quality of Life**

Tip: Focus on the positive aspects of maintaining kidney health. Discover new, tasty recipes and explore enjoyable activities that align with your dietary needs.

7. **Concern: Social Isolation**

Tip: Educate friends and family about your renal diet. Encourage open conversations about your dietary needs to avoid feeling isolated during meals together.

8. **Concern: Dietary Monotony**

Tip: Vary your meals by trying new fruits, vegetables, and protein sources. Experiment with different cooking techniques to keep your diet interesting.

9. **Concern: Difficulty Dining Out**

Tip: Call restaurants ahead of time to discuss your dietary needs. Many establishments are willing to accommodate special requests or offer alternatives.

10. **Concern: Impact on Mental Health**

Tip: Seek support from healthcare professionals, support groups, or mental health experts. Focus on maintaining a positive mindset and finding joy in your dietary choices.

11. **Concern: Protein Intake**

Tip: Collaborate with a dietitian to plan a balanced diet that meets your protein needs without overloading your kidneys. Explore plant-based protein sources.

12. **Concern: Balancing Multiple Health Conditions**

Tip: Establish a healthcare team that includes specialists for each health condition. Ensure open communication among healthcare professionals for a comprehensive care plan.

13. **Concern: Misinformation**

Tip: Rely on trusted sources of information, such as healthcare professionals and reputable renal health organizations. Consult with a registered dietitian for personalized advice.

Remember, troubleshooting concerns related to a renal diet requires ongoing communication with healthcare professionals. Regular check-ins with your healthcare team and adjustments to your dietary plan can help address specific challenges and optimize your kidney health.

CONCLUSION

In conclusion, embracing a renal-friendly lifestyle is a journey toward improved kidney health and overall well-being. Through commitment to a balanced renal diet, adherence to prescribed medications, and proactive engagement with healthcare professionals, individuals can navigate the challenges of managing kidney health successfully. Celebrating progress, fostering a positive mindset, and staying connected to support networks are integral aspects of this journey.

Whether it's making mindful dietary choices, incorporating regular physical activity, or practicing stress management, each step contributes to the goal of maintaining optimal kidney function. The commitment to kidney-friendly living extends beyond individual efforts; it involves collaboration with healthcare professionals, social support networks, and a continuous pursuit of knowledge about renal health.

By acknowledging achievements, cultivating resilience, and fostering adaptability, individuals can thrive on the path to kidney-friendly living. The dedication to a balanced lifestyle not only supports renal health but also empowers individuals to lead fulfilling lives. With gratitude for progress made and a commitment to ongoing self-care, the journey toward renal well-being becomes a transformative and empowering experience.